Aromatherapy

How to use natures remedies to improve your health and wellbeing

Faye Froome

Contents

Introduction

I want to thank you for purchasing the book, *Aromatherapy – How to use natures remedies to improve your health and wellbeing.*

This book contains information on how use what nature provides to heal and strengthen your mind and body.

Study the secrets of aromatherapy; discover the history of an ancient practice which has been used successfully for centuries; learn how to apply it to your life and how to benefit both physically and mentally from its use.

You will also find recipes which will enable you to create soaps, skin care products and much more which you can adapt to suit your body or give as gifts to friends and family.

So what are you waiting for, turn the page and discover a natural way to improve your life.

Thanks again for purchasing this book; I really hope you enjoy it!

Chapter 1 – What Are Essential Oils

Essential oils are the complete essence of a plant and contain no added ingredients. The leaves, flowers, stems, roots, bark, in fact any part of a plant can be used to make essential oil. Simply put, they are the very spirit of the plant that has been extracted and bottled.

An essential oil contains all the qualities of the plant in a highly concentrated form and, as such, they are extremely potent. One or two drops of pure oil will require a large amount of the plant to produce it. To put this into perspective, (and I use this as a hypothetical example only to show the ratio), 2 drops of oil made from a tea plant would require more of the plant than is found in a full box of teabags.

Essential oils are usually sold in small bottles and appear to contain very little product in comparison to the cost however, when the small quantities of oil required for each use is taken into consideration, most oils prove to be very reasonably priced. Additionally, the oils have a long use by date so are not limited to use by a time scale.

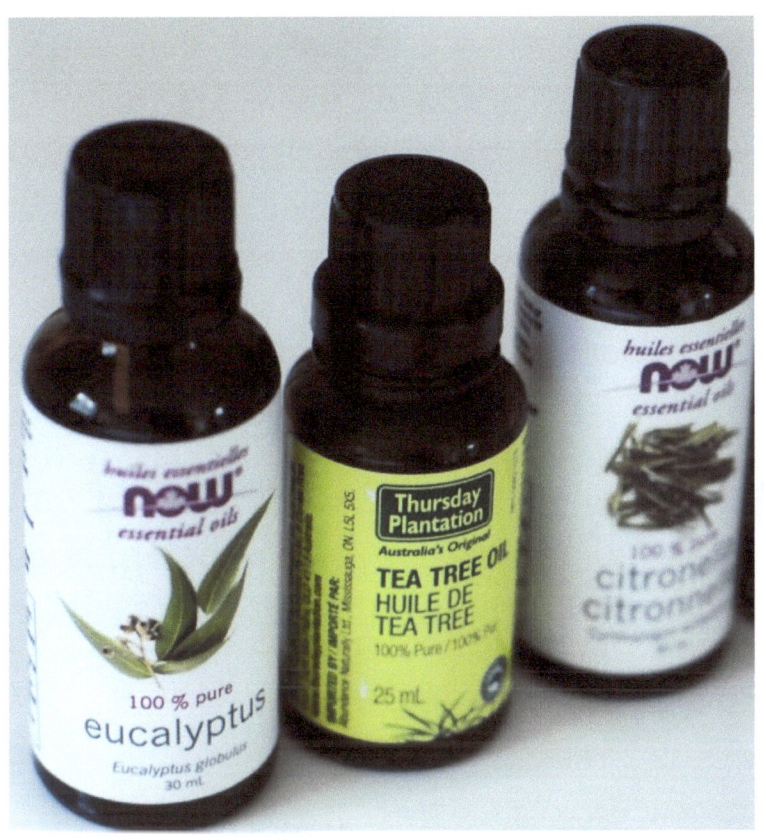

There is not just one type of aromatherapy oil so it is important to understand the differences. Many lower priced aromatherapy oils on the market have no therapeutic benefits.

Any oil marked with the words perfume or fragrance is not an essential oil, they will make your room smell pleasant, but will offer no health benefit. In contrast, an essential oil will have a psychological and/or physiological effect on the mind and/or body.

Unlike a manufactured medicinal product such as medicine or tablets, essential oils cause no build up within the body. They are completely natural and are fully absorbed, they then travel through the body doing their job before they pass out of you leaving no residue.

The majority of oils contain one or more properties which include:

- Anti-viral

- Anti-bacterial

- Anti-fungal

These properties allow for versatility in the use of the oils and they can be used to make everything from skin care to cleaning products. However you use them, because of their amazing qualities you are sure to gain health benefits.

Essential oils are made by extracting the useful properties of the plant by using, most commonly, steam or water methods. This type of extraction is used to produce the majority of oils on the market however, other methods are sometimes used and each method produces slightly different results.

The oils obtained through different extractions are known as Absolutes and CO2s.
Absolutes: Extracted using a solvent method which produces a higher concentration of plant molecules making absolutes considerably stronger than other essential oils.

CO2's: Extracted using a pressurized form of carbon dioxide. CO2 oils are often thicker than oils made using other methods. They also retain a higher level of the plants natural aroma.

Chapter 2 – Origins of Aromatherapy

During the 20th century aromatherapy grew in popularity and its wide spread use became increasingly common. This was largely due to the efforts of a French chemist named Rene-Maurice Gattefosse who, during the 1930's accidentally discovered the benefits of lavender oil.

Whilst carrying out work in his laboratory, Rene-Maurice burnt his hand and reacted instinctively by plunging it straight into the nearest vat of liquid. As luck would have it, the vat contained lavender oil. Surprised by how quickly the burn healed and the fact that no scarring was evident, Gattefosse began to intensively study the beneficial effects of essential oils.

This study led to him producing what is reputedly the first published work on the subject of aromatherapy in 1937. 'Aromatherapie: Les Huilles Essentialles'. This was followed by a post world war 2 publication of a book entitled 'The Practice of Aromatherapy' written by Dr. Jean Valnet who had included the practical use of essential oils when treating injured soldiers during the war.

In 1977, world famous aromatherapist, Robert B Tisserand wrote 'The Art of Aromatherapy'. This was the first book on the subject to be written and published in English. Since then the interest in the use of essential oils has continued to grow.

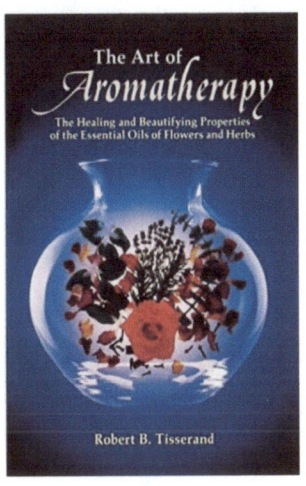

While it may appear that aromatherapy is a relatively modern concept, its roots are firmly based thousands of years ago with the Ancient Egyptians who are recognized as being the earliest known practitioners in the use of essential oils.

According to research, the embalming of bodies prior to mummification was originally used (2650 – 2575 BC). The practitioners believed that the use of essential oils on the bodies of their dead royalty would preserve the body during its journey into the afterlife.

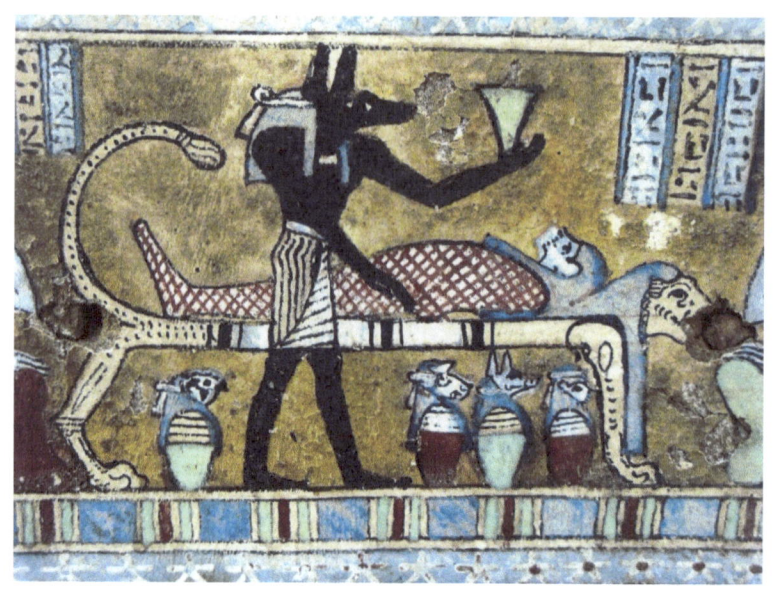

By 657 BC the use of essential oils had progressed to include use on the living as well as the dead. Many oils were utilized in the treatment of ailments, as incense and for perfume and cosmetics.

Later Hippocrates (460 – 370BC), often referred to as the 'Father of Medicine', began to study the healing benefits and beneficial uses of essential oils.

More recently, during the scourge of the Black Death in the 14th century, it is widely believed that the reason many perfumers didn't contract the disease was due to their work with essential oils.

Chapter 3 – How to Use Essential Oils

There are a variety of different methods for applying the use of essential oils to your life. Whether you are treating a specific ailment or using the oils for an all round boost, you will find the process to be relaxing and easy to implement.

- Inhaling oils offers the psychological benefits attributed to the particular oil you are using in addition to the physiological benefit received by inhaling the oil directly into your lungs.

- Skin application allows the oil to be quickly absorbed through the skin and into the blood stream.

There are very few oils which are safe to apply directly to the skin so they will need to be diluted. Carrier oils such as almond oil, is the most common substance used for diluting essential oils as they facilitate the distribution of the essential oils without hindering their benefits.

Many oils can be bought pre-diluted if you prefer however, if you would rather do this yourself using the pure oil then typically the average amount of essential oil to carrier ratio is 2%, e.g. 10 – 12 drops of oil to 30ml of carrier oil.

CAUTION: This amount is a recommendation only. As absolutes are far more concentrated than regular oils this amount should be at least halved. The quality of the oils should also be considered when diluting. Quality cannot be based on price however as there is a large difference in the cost of production in varying oils. The amount of plant required to produce the oil can be significantly different between plants. For therapeutic benefits always choose a grade 'A' oil. The lower the plant grade, the lower the oil quality.

Some essential oils have properties that can also be used in insect repellents and cleaning products.

In addition to physical treatment, the scent of many oils causes a psychological reaction within the brain which has a positive effect on the mood helping to lift and energize. There has also been much progress in scientific research in this area with positive findings which show that certain aromatherapy oils can aid mental ability, with improvements being shown in both memory and concentration.

Many mental and physical problems have a number of symptoms so it can be useful to blend 2 or more oils together to aid all areas of a problem rather than treating each symptom separately.

Carrier Oils

Carrier oils are predominantly made from the seeds, nuts and kernels of vegetables. Unlike essential oils, carrier oils can become unusable due to fatty acids they contain. Most carriers have only a mild scent so if you discover your carrier has a particularly strong and unpleasant smell it should be discarded.

Natural vegetable based creams, lotions and balms can also be used as carriers if you prefer and these are particularly useful in skin care products. Cocoa butter and Shea butter can also be used for this purpose.

There are many different vegetable oils on the market. My 2 favorite carriers are:

Sweet Almond Oil; affordable and easily absorbed into the skin. This is perfect for use as a carrier for massage oil. Avoid if you suffer from nut allergies.

Grapeseed Oil; Affordable and absorbs well but often leaves a light coating on the skin. I find this works well for almost any skin application of essential oil. This oil has a limited shelf life of around 6 – 12 months.

Methods of Use

PLEASE NOTE: Recommended drops of oil are not the pure oil but oil that has been mixed with a carrier oil.

Steam Inhalation

This method is particularly useful for the treatment of respiratory problems, colds, flu and sinus problems but it is not limited to these conditions. With the right oils, steam inhalation also works wonders for relaxation in the evening or for gaining an energy boost during the day.

Pour 1 to 2 pints of boiling water into a bowl and add 3- 4 drops of essential oil. (1 -2 drops of an absolute).

Place your head over the bowl and cover head and bowl with a towel.

Breathe in deeply through nose or mouth to inhale the steam. This ensures the oil reaches your lungs in a very short time and will begin to treat any problems or viruses quickly and effectively.

Inhalation

This is a quick and easy way to treat problems when you are out and about. Place 2 – 4 drops of oil onto a handkerchief or other small piece of material and inhale deeply through mouth or nose. If you are using the oil to aid sleep and relaxation, a few drops can be placed onto the corner of your bed sheet or pillowcase.

Massage

This is a very pleasant and relaxing way of using essential oils. Not only does a gentle massage soothe tired achy muscles but it also aids the circulatory system and nervous system. By adding essential oil, or blend of oils, to your carrier the oils are absorbed into your skin and aid healing and health. Add 3 – 5 drops of essential oil per 10ml of almond oil.

Massage with essential oils is not restricted to adults. Although many oils are not suitable for children and babies, there are a few that are.

1 drop of lavender oil can be added to a bottle of baby oil to make relaxing massage oil for babies. When massaging babies, use only very gentle stroking motions on their skin. This is great to do straight after a bath and before bed.

Bathing

Adding oils to your bath is one of the easiest ways to absorb therapeutic oils into your skin, and the scent of most oils will add to the relaxing atmosphere of your bathroom.

Mix 6 – 8 drops of essential oil into a natural bath oil or carrier oil and stir into your bath. Oils can be added directly to the bath water but it is unlikely they will be absorbed properly into your skin as they will float on the surface of the water.

Foot Bath

To refresh tired, aching feet after a hard day, add 3 -4 drops of oil to a large bowl of warm water and soak your feet for 10 – 15 minutes.

This method can be used effectively to treat other ailments that are unrelated to your feet, depending on the oil you use, and is a relaxing way to use essential oils.

Compress

Hot or cold compresses should be used for a maximum of 20 minutes at a time.

For either hot or cold compresses, add 4 – 5 drops of oil to your water, (ice cold or hot). Mix in and soak a flannel in the water for a couple of minutes. Wring out flannel and apply to relevant area.

Hot compress; period pain, arthritis, joint pain or muscle cramps.

Cold compress; sprains, inflammation, bruising and headache.

Gargling
DO NOT SWALLOW

For sore throats, mouth ulcers or gum problems add 1 drop of essential oil to a cup of water and gargle for a maximum of 30 seconds before spitting. Wait five to ten minutes then gargle and spit with plain water.

Burning

Oil burners and candles are an effective way to reap the beneficial effects of essential oils and make your room smell lovely.

This works on the inhalation method but is much less intense as the oil is not being inhaled directly into your system from close proximity, however, for preventative treatments this is an easy way to keep on top of your ailments.

For burners, add 2 -3 drops of oil to a little water. Candles can be used by rubbing a few drops of mixed essential and carrier oil onto your palms and rubbing your hands along the outside of a candle before lighting it. This keeps the oils away from the flame but allows them to be dispersed into the air as the wax heats.

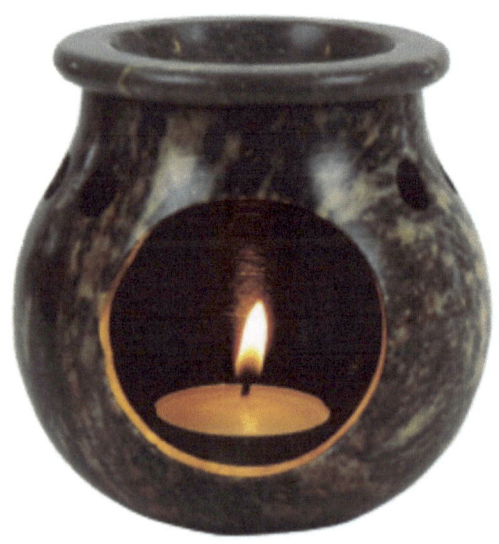

Skin Products

Natural, unscented soaps, moisturizers and lotions are a great way to incorporate essential oils into your hygiene or beauty routine. Add 2 – 3 drops of oil into your carrier and apply daily. Not only will this be good for your skin but it will provide a daily dose of oil to treat any relevant health problems.

Household Uses

For freshening up your home add a couple of drops of essential oil to your vacuum filter. The heat generated by the appliance when it is being used will help the scent to spread around your home as you are cleaning.

When using a tumble dryer, add a few drops of your chosen oil to a clean, dry handkerchief and place in the tumble dryer with your wet laundry.

Many natural cleaning products can be made using essential oils and soaps. (See recipe section)

Chapter 4 – Safety & Essential Oils

You should not assume that because essential oils are completely natural they can be used in large amounts or that they are safe for everyone to use. Even vitamin and mineral tablets can make you very ill if they are taken in incorrect dosages so caution MUST be used with oils. That said, when used correctly they are a safe and pleasant way to heal yourself and prevent illnesses.

Due to the high concentration of properties contained within essential oils they can be extremely dangerous is too much is used so always pay close attention to the directions on the bottle.

Always treat essential oils with the same respect you would give to a prescribed medication.

The oils listed below should never be used as they are toxic:
- **Parsley**
- **Pennyroyal**
- **Savin**
- **Tansy**
- **Wintergreen**
- **Wormwood**

Pregnancy

There are many oils which are safe to use when pregnant but before using you should seek advice from your midwife, a qualified health care advisor or a professional homeopathic aromatherapy practitioner.

You may also find that some oils which are safe to use, and which you have used successfully in the past, will cause adverse reactions now you are pregnant. This is due to the changes in your hormone levels.

Some oils should never be used on or around a pregnant woman as they can cause serious complications with the pregnancy and have unwanted repercussions.

If pregnant or breast feeding do not use:
- Aniseed
- Angelica
- Basil
- Birch
- Black Pepper
- Camphor
- Chamomile
- Clary Sage

- Clove
- Fennel
- Fir
- Ginger
- Horseradish
- Hyssup
- Jasmine
- Juniper
- Marjoram
- Mustard
- Mugwort
- Myrrh
- Nutmeg
- Oregano
- Parsley
- Pennyroyal
- Peppermint
- Rosemary
- Sage
- Tansy
- Tarragon
- Thuja
- Thyme
- Wintergreen
- Wormwood

Babies & Children

Many oils are unsuitable for use on babies and young children. The essential that can be used should be less than adult dosage. Once children are above six years old and over, most adult use oils are safe to use in lesser amounts.

Use one third of an adult dosage for children aged between 6 and 10, (unless they are of a very small build, in which case stick to the under 5 years of age recommendations).

Ages 11 to 15 use a half adult dosage.

The recommended amount of essential oil for children under 5 years of age and babies is based on weight.

Weight

6 – 12 kilograms (13.2 lb – 26.4 lb) = 1 drop of diluted oil
12 – 25 kilograms (26.4 lb – 55.1 lb) = 2 – 3 drops of diluted oil
25 – 38 kilograms (55.1 lb – 83.7 lb) = 4 – 5 drops of diluted oil

Avoid these oils for babies & toddlers aged 3 years old and younger (Before using any oil, other than lavender on a baby, check with a midwife or health advisor).

- Basil
- Bay
- Cassia
- Cinnamon Bark
- Citronella
- Citrus
- Clove
- Fennel
- Lemongrass
- Mugwort
- Oregano
- Thyme
- And all listed for avoidance for 5 years and under

Children under 5 years old avoid

- Bergamot
- Birch
- Tansy
- Nutmeg
- Peppermint
- Rosemary
- Sage
- Spearmint
- Tarragon
- Wintergreen

Medication & Illness

Some illnesses and medications can produce an adverse reaction to certain oils. While there is much debate as to the number of oils which should be avoided, some oils have been listed consistently as proving to be detrimental to various conditions.

Below are the most frequently recommended oils to avoid however, if you are taking any regular medication for an ongoing problem, or have any of the conditions listed below I would advise you seek advice from a healthcare/holistic practitioner before using essential oils.

Advice should always be sought before using:
- Dill
- Fennel
- Nutmeg

If you suffer from high blood pressure you should avoid:
- Hyssop
- Rosemary
- Sage
- Thyme

If you suffer with epilepsy you should avoid:
- Basil
- Birch
- Hyssop
- Tansy
- Rosemary
- Sage
- Tarragon
- Wintergreen

Diabetics should avoid:
- Angelica

When taking anti-coagulant drugs you should avoid:
- Birch
- Clove
- Ginger
- Wintergreen

The following oils should not be used consistently for more than 2 weeks:
- Aniseed
- Cinnamon
- Coriander
- Eucalyptus
- Laurel
- Juniper
- Turmeric
- Valerian

Photo-toxicity

UV light can cause problems to occur with some oils when they are exposed to it. This can result in changes to skin pigmentation which varies from mild to deep color change and mild to severe burning of the skin.

If you plan on using a sun bed, sunbathing or spending time outdoors on particular sunny day you should avoid the following essential oils for 48 hours prior to the exposure of skin to UV rays.

- Angelica
- Bergamot
- Cumin
- Grapefruit
- Lemon
- Lime
- Orange
- Taget
- Rue

Sensitization

Sensitization is similar to an allergic reaction and can cause itching, inflammation, redness and, in some cases, sore skin. The first sign of sensitization developing with particular oils should feel like only a minor irritation, however, continued use of the particular oil will result in the irritation developing into a stronger reaction.

Some oils are more prone to causing sensitization than others so it is advised that the following oils be used for a maximum of 3 to 4 days before having a few days break from them to help avoid this.
- Bay
- Cassia
- Cinnamon
- Clove
- Origanum
- Thyme
- Tagette

General Safety Advice

- Never swallow any essential oil

- Essential oils are flammable so always store oils out of direct sunlight and away from naked flames

- Always dilute oils before using directly on the skin. (Some oils are safe to use without dilution but there are very few that are this safe so unless advised by a profession practitioner of aromatherapy avoid all oils being used in this way)

- Perform a sensitivity test before using any new variety of oil. Dilute 1 drop of essential oil in 1 teaspoon of carrier oil and apply to the inner forearm. If no adverse reaction has occurred within 3 hours the oil should be safe to use.

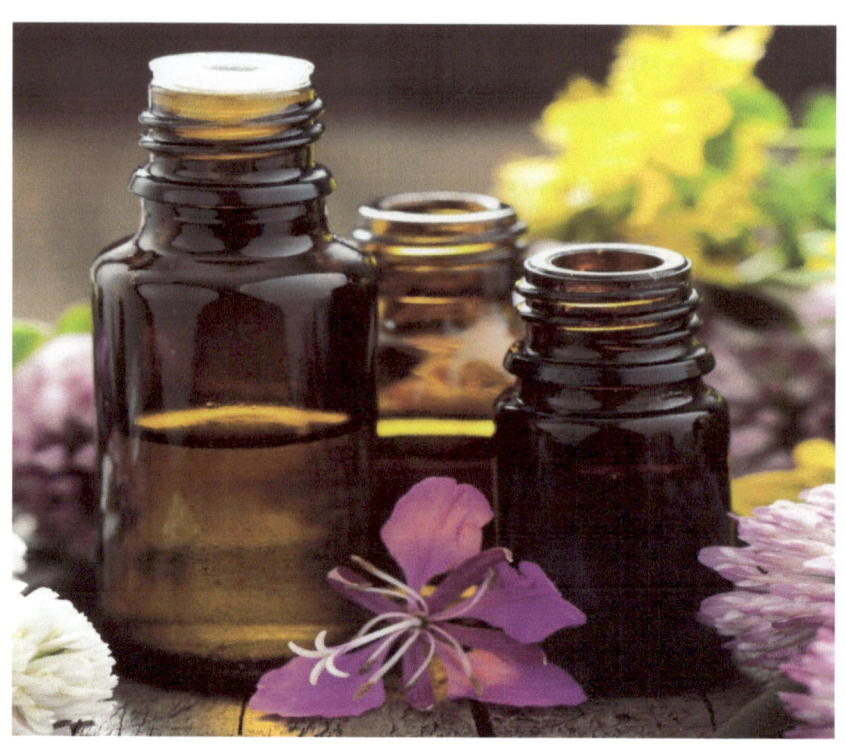

Chapter 5 – Recipes Using Essential Oils

This chapter contains recipes for making your own health and skincare products. To personalize the recipes for your own needs, change the oil or blend of oils to suit your skin type, skin condition, mood requirements, physical condition or psychological requirement.

Oils to suit skin type or skin condition

Normal Skin: Lavender, Geranium, Ylang-Ylang, Jasmine, Chamomile, Neroli
Oily Skin: Sandalwood, Lemon, Lavender, Geranium, Chamomile, Cedarwood
Dry Skin: Sandalwood, Geranium, Rose, Jasmine, Orange, Rosewood
Combination Skin: Geranium, Rose Geranium, Neroli, Rosewood, Ylang Ylang
Sensitive Skin: Chamomile, Rose, Neroli, Jasmine
Mature Skin: Neroli, Frankincense, Ylang-Ylang , Geranium, Myrrh,
Acne: Lemon, Cypress, Lavender, Geranium, Patchouli, Tea Tree
Broken capillaries: Rose, Chamomile, Cypress

Eczema: Myrrh, Patchouli, Lavender, Bergamot, Sandalwood, German Chamomile, Tea Tree, Cedarwood, Ylang Ylang

Scars & Stretch Marks: Frankincense, Geranium, Lavender, Rose

Chapped Skin: Lavender, Sandalwood, Chamomile, Myrrh, Patchouli, Sandalwood

Itching: Jasmine, Lavender, Chamomile, peppermint

To Re-Hydrate Skin: Rose, Sandalwood, Patchoulli

To Revitalise Skin: Geranium, Rose, Cypress

Cleansing: Juniper, Sweet Basil, Lemongrass, Peppermint, Lemon

Toning: Chamomile, Lavender, Neroli, Rose, Organge, Frankincense, Petigrain, Lemon, Lemongrass

Carrier Oils for skin care:

Dry Skin and/or Night Treatments: Jojoba Oil - Easily absorbed into skin but leaves a light covering of oil on the skins surface

Alternatives for Dry Skin: Sweet Almond Oil, Avocado Oil

Oily Skin and/or Daytime Treatments: Rosehip Oil - Dry oil that absorbs easily into skin and is full of skin boosting properties

Alternatives for Oily Skin: Grapeseed Oil

Eczema/Psoriasis Treatments: Hemp Seed Oil – very dry oil which won't clog up the pores. This oil has produced excellent effects in the treatment of eczema and psoriasis. This oil contains no THC's which are associated with the cannabis plant.

Exfoliating Body Scrubs

Body Scrub 1
Ingredients:
- 1 cup castor sugar
- ¼ cup carrier oil
- 2 tbsp raw honey
- 15 - 20 drops essential oil(s) of your choice

Body Scrub 2
Ingredients:
- 1 cup brown sugar (finely ground)
- $1/3$ cup carrier oil
- 15 – 20 drops essential oil(s) of your choice

Body Scrub 3
Ingredients:
- 1 cup salt (finely ground)
- $1/3$ cup carrier oil
- 15 – 20 drops essential oil(s) of your choice

Preparation:
1. Add all ingredients to a bowl and mix together well.

2. Store in an airtight container and away from natural sunlight.

Foot Scrubs

Foot Scrub 1
Ingredients:
- 1 cup salt
- $^1/_3$ cup carrier oil
- 15 drops essential oil(s) of your choice

Foot Scrub 2
Ingredients:
- 1 cup brown sugar
- 1/3 cup carrier oil
- 12 – 15 drops essential oil(s) of your choice

Preparation:
1. Add all ingredients to a bowl and mix together well.

2. Store in an airtight container and away from natural sunlight.

Bath Salts

Ingredients:

- 1 cup sea salt
- 2 tbsp bicarbonate of soda
- 1 cup epsom salts
- 12 – 15 drops essential oil(s) of your choice

Preparation:

1. Mix together sea salt and Epsom salts
2. Sieve bicarbonate of soda and stir into salt mix
3. Add essential oil(s) and mix well

To Use:

Pour ½ cup of bath salts into running water and stir into bath
Store in an airtight container and away from natural sunlight

Bath Bombs

Ingredients:
- 1 cup citric acid or ½ cup cream of tartar
- 1 tbsp carrier oil
- 2 cups baking soda
- ½ - 1 tsp water
- 20 - 25 drops essential oil(s) of your choice
- Bath bomb molds

Bath Bomb Molds:

Bath bombs do not have to be round so if you can't get hold of a ball shaped mold, improvise. Plastic balls cut into halves make a great substitute for round molds. Alternatively, consider what you have in your home already. Muffin tins or trays, chocolate molds, small jelly molds, shot glasses or even cookie cutters are all useful and make interestingly shaped bath bombs.

It is helpful if you cover the inside of your molds with cling film to aid in removing them without breaking.

Preparation:
1. Mix together citric acid, baking soda and carrier oil

2. Add essential oils and mix together well

3. If mixture is too powdery add water, 1 drop at a time, and mix. Water MUST be added slowly and stirred in gently to avoid it reacting with the other ingredients before you are ready to use it. Alternatively, you can add an additional drop or two of carrier oil.

Why not experiment by adding a few drops of food coloring or some chopped petals.

Foaming Facial Wash

Ingredients:
1 cup cooled, boiled water
¼ cup liquid castile soap
5 tsp carrier oil
2 tbsp raw honey
5 drops tea tree oil
15 drops essential oil(s) of your choice

Preparation:
1. Pour water into a bowl and slowly stir in the castile soap

2. Add carrier oil and raw honey and gently mix together

3. Add essential oils and stir together

4. Gently pour soap into liquid soap dispenser

Use 1 – 2 pumps of soap at a time
Ingredients may separate so give dispenser a gentle shake as needed

Exfoliating Facial Wash

Recipe makes enough facial wash for 1 use
Ingredients:
½ tbsp lemon juice
½ tbsp water
2 tbsp baking soda
3 drops of essential oil(s) of your choice

Preparation:
1. Mix together lemon juice, water and baking soda

2. Add essential oils and stir into a paste

To Use:
1. Apply paste to face and gently massage into the skin for 1 – 2 minutes

2. Rinse with warm water and pat dry

Soap Bars

Recipe makes 8 – 12 bars of soap
Ingredients:
- ¼ cup coconut oil
- ¼ cup shea butter
- ¼ cup beeswax, (grated)
- 50 drops essential oil(s) of your choice
- Optional: 3 drops vitamin E oil

Preparation:
1. Place a heat proof bowl over a pan of simmering water on the stove

2. Add beeswax, coconut oil and shea butter to the bowl and stir until melted and mix together

3. Remove bowl from heat and add vitamin E (if using) and essential oils

4. Stir together well and pour mixture into molds

Alternatively you can pour the mixture onto a shallow baking tray and cut soap to size when set Soap bars have a shelf life of up to 6 months. Store in a cool place out of direct sunlight

Body Butter

Ingredients:
- ¼ cup coconut oil
- ¼ cup carrier oil
- ½ cup shea butter
- 8 – 10 drops essential oil(s) of your choice

Preparation:
1. Place a heat proof bowl over a pan of simmering water on the stove

2. Add shea butter, carrier oil and coconut oil to the bowl and stir together until melted (mixture will fade from white and become clearer)

3. Remove from heat and allow mixture to cool for 1 hour, mixture will solidify as it cools

4. Once cooled, use a blender or electric mixer to beat the solidified mixture. Continue to beat the mix until fluffy. (You can do this by hand but it will take much longer)

5. Add essential oils and stir well

6. Pour mix into a container or mold and place in the fridge for an hour to set

Cleansing Serum

Ingredients:
- 2 oz Coconut oil

- 5 – 6 drops essential oil(s) of your choice

Preparation:
1. Mix together coconut oil and essential oil

2. Apply to face and massage into skin for up to 1 minute

3. Remove with a warm, damp flannel

Use once or twice per week

Alternative Oil:
Argon oil is a good alternative to coconut oil, or you can use a combination of the two,
Argon oil contains vitamins C and E. The antioxidant properties of these vitamins are great for all ages and skin types but work particularly well on mature skin as they can aid the elasticity of the skin.

Skin Toner

Ingredients:

- 8 fl oz cooled, boiled water

Essential Oils

- 2 drops lavender oil
  1 drop palmarosa oil
  1 drop rosewood oil

Preparation:

1. Mix together all ingredients and shake well

To Use:

Apply to face using a cotton wool boil

Store in a dark coloured, airtight container away from direct sunlight

Shampoo

Ingredients:
- ½ cup liquid castile soap
- ½ tsp vegetable glycerin
- 5 – 8 drops of essential oil(s) of your choice

Preparation:
1. Mix together all ingredients

Store in a dark, airtight container away from direct sunlight

Mood Blends

Energising: grapefruit, bergamot, peppermint

Detoxifying: grapefruit, lemon, juniper

Relaxing: sandalwood, neroli, rose

Romantic: orange, patchoulli, cinnamon, ylang ylang

Soothing: lavender, mandarin

Essential Oils for Men

When we think of essential oils and their use in everyday life, most people assume they are restricted mainly to women due to their feminine scents. Below is a list of essential oils that have a more masculine scent and can be used in the manufacture of male skin care and fragrance products.

- Bay Laurel
- Bergamot
- Cedar
- Clary Sage
- Cypress
- Fir
- Frankincense
- Juniper Berry
- Lemon Balm
- Lime
- Myrrh
- Neroli
- Oakmoss
- Orange
- Sage
- Sandalwood
- Spruce
- Thyme
- Tobacco
- Vetiver

Aftershave balm

Make your man a soothing and healing aftershave balm that not only smells great but has therapeutic properties to relieve anxiety or symptoms of stress.

Balm Recipe 1

This recipe makes enough balm for 2 or 3 days

Ingredients:
- 1 tsp coconut oil
- 1 drop lemongrass
- 1 drop cedarwood
- 1 drop lavender

Preparation:
1. Mix together all ingredients

Store in an airtight container away from direct sunlight

For a more personalized scent you can replace the lemongrass and cedarwood oils. Mix and match with the suggested masculine scented oils to achieve a balm which will appeal to the man wearing it.

Balm Recipe 2

Ingredients:
- 1 cup witch hazel
- 1 tsp vegetable glycerin
- 6 drops orange
- 3 drops sandalwood

Preparation:

Mix together all ingredients and store in a dark coloured bottle out of direct sunlight

Rub a couple of drops onto your hands and pat onto shaved area

Skin replenishing oil

This blend is perfect for replenishing the facial skin during times of stress, insomnia or after a heavy night on the town.

Ingredients:
- 4 tbsp carrier oil or coconut oil
- 10 drops bergamot
- 5 drops patchouli

Preparation:

1. Mix all ingredients together and apply a thin layer to skin

Store in an airtight container away from direct sunlight

Moisturising Facial Scrub
Ingredients:

- 1 teaspoon water
- 2 tsp carrier oil
- 1 tsp honey
- 5 drops of essential oil(s) of your choice
- 2 tbsp ground oatmeal
- 1/4 teaspoon sea salt (finely ground)

Preparation:
Combine all ingredients and mix together into a paste. If a little too thick ad a few extra drops of water

Apply to the face and massage in for 1 minute

Rinse with warm water and pat dry

Fragrance Oils for Men

For fragrance oils you can choose to use firm oils such as coconut oil or liquid oils such as almond or jojoba. If you prefer to use liquid oils, a thinner variety is preferable to the heavier, thick carrier oils.

To make 20ml of liquid use 4 teaspoons of carrier oil

For a firmer fragrance oil use 4 teaspoons of coconut oil

Always store fragrance oils in a dark container and away from direct sunlight

A few dabs of these fragrances should be enough to last several hours

Relaxing Fragrance Oil

- 2 drops patchouli
- 4 drops cedarwood
- 4 drops sandalwood

Energising Fragrance Oil

- 4 drops sandalwood
- 4 drops lime
- 2 drops ginger

To Aid Concentration

- 4 drops rosemary
- 4 drops lemon
- 2 drops peppermint

Evening Fragrance Oil

- 1 drop cedarwood
- 1 drop ylang ylang
- 8 drops grapefruit

Essential Oils Blends for Common Ailments

Blends to Ease Stress

Bath Oil
Makes enough oil for 7 – 8 baths
Ingredients:
- 60 ml carrier oil
- 9 drops bergamot
- 3 drops frankincense
- 3 drops geranium

Preparation:
Blend ingredients together and add to bath under running water.

Massage Oil
Ingredients:
- 30 ml carrier oil
- 6 drops grapefruit
- 2 drops ylang ylang
- 2 drops jasmine

Preparation:
Mix together ingredients and place in a dark, airtight bottle.
Store in a cool place out of direct sunlight

Blends to Ease Anxiety

Bath Oil
Makes enough oil for 7 – 8 baths
Ingredients:
- 60 ml carrier oil

- 6 drops mandarin

- 3 drops rose

- 3 drops vetiver

- 3 drops lavender

Preparation:
Blend ingredients together and add to bath under running water.

Massage Oil
Ingredients:
- 30 ml carrier oil

- 6 drops sandalwood

- 4 drops bergamot

Preparation:
Mix together ingredients and place in a dark, airtight bottle.
Store in a cool place out of direct sunlight

Blends to Ease Depression

Bath Oil
Makes enough oil for 7 – 8 baths
Ingredients:
- 60 ml carrier oil

- 6 drops neroli

- 6 drops frankincense

- 3 drops lemon

Preparation:
Blend ingredients together and add to bath under running water.

Massage Oil
Ingredients:
- 30 ml carrier oil

- 6 drops sandalwood

- 2 drops rose

- 2 drops orange

Preparation:
Mix together ingredients and place in a dark, airtight bottle.
Store in a cool place out of direct sunlight

Blends to Ease Headaches & Migraines

Bath Oil
Makes enough oil for 7 – 8 baths
Ingredients:
- 60 ml carrier oil

- 7 drops peppermint

- 5 drops eucalyptus

- 3 drops Myrrh

Preparation:
Blend ingredients together and add to bath under running water.

Massage Oil
Ingredients:
- 30 ml carrier oil

- 6 drops peppermint

- 2 drops eucalyptus

- 2 drops lavendar

Preparation:
Mix together ingredients and place in a dark, airtight bottle.
Store in a cool place out of direct sunlight

Chapter 6 – Index: Uses of Essential Oils

This chapter contains an index of common ailments and the beneficial oils which can be used to treat them.

These oils can be used in skin products, massage oils, burners and all other practical application methods.

When choosing your oils consider all symptoms relating to the problem you are treating. Use oils either separately or in a blend to achieve the maximum benefit.

Abdominal Pain

- Peppermint
- Ginger
- Chamomile
- Cumin

Acne

- Tea Tree
- Lavender
- Frankincense
- Geranium
- Clary Sage
- Chamomile
- Oregano
- Ylang Ylang
- Bergamot
- Lemongrass

Anxiety

- Bergamot
- Basil
- Chamomile
- Clary Sage
- Frankincense
- Geranium
- Jasmine
- Lemon
- Lavender

- Mandarin
- Marjoram
- Orange
- Palmarosa
- Rose
- Sandalwood
- Ylang Ylang

Athletes Foot

- Clove
- Eucalyptus
- Geranium
- Lavender
- Lemongrass
- Myrrh
- Peppermint
- Sandalwood
- Tea Tree
- Thyme

Bruises

- Arnica
- Cypress
- Geranium
- Lavender
- Lemongrass
- Myrrh
- Rosemary

Burns

- Frankincense
- Lavender
- Peppermint
- Tea Tree

Catarhh

- Eucalyptus
- Lanvender
- Peppermint
- Tea Tree

Circulation Problems

- Basil
- Clove
- Grapefruit
- Lemon
- Marjoram
- Neroli
- Rosemary
- Thyme

Coldsores

- Lavender
- Lemon Balm
- Tea Tree

Colds & Flu

- Eucalyptus
- Lavender
- Lemon
- Peppermint
- Pine
- Rosemary
- Tea Tree

- Thyme

Constipation

- Ginger
- Lemon
- Marjoram
- Orange
- Peppermint
- Rose
- Rosemary
- Sweet Basil

Coughs

- Angelica
- Black Pepper
- Cedarwood
- Cypress
- Eucalyptus
- Frankincense

- Lavender
- Lemon
- Myrrh
- Peppermint
- Rosemary
- Sandalwood
- Tea Tree

Cuts & Grazes

- Clary Sage
- Eucalyptus
- Frankincense
- Geranium
- Grapefruit
- Juniper
- Lavender
- Lemon
- Myrrh
- Orange
- Oregano
- Patchouli
- Peppermint
- Pine
- Sandalwood
- Tea Tree
- Thyme
- Ylang Ylang

Depression

- Bergamot
- Basil
- Cedarwood
- Clary Sage
- Frankincense
- Geranium
- Grapefruit
- Lavender
- Lemon
- Jasmine
- Myrrh
- Neroli
- Orange
- Rose
- Sandalwood
- Spruce
- Ylang Ylang

Diarrhea

- Basil
- Chamomile
- Coriander
- Dill
- Frankincense
- Ginger
- Lavender
- Lemon

- Marjoram
- Orange
- Peppermint
- Tangerine
- Tea Tree

Fatigue

- Basil
- Bergamot
- Grapefruit
- Lemon
- Neroli
- Orange
- Peppermint
- Petigrain
- Spearmint

Fever

- Lavender
- Peppermint

Gingivitis

- Clove
- Cinnamon
- Myrrh
- Peppermint
- Spearmint

Hay Fever
- Chamomile
- Clove
- Eucalyptus
- Lavender

- Lemon
- Peppermint

Headaches
- Chamomile
- Eucalyptus
- Lavender
- Peppermint
- Spearmint

Immune System
- Bay
- Bergamot
- Chamomile
- Cinnamon
- Eucalyptus
- Frankincense
- Lavender
- Laurel
- Myrrh
- Oregano
- Pine

- Sage
- Sandalwood
- Tea Tree
- Thyme
- Vetiver

Insect Bites
- Basil
- Eucalyptus
- Lavender
- Peppermint
- Rosemary
- Tea Tree
- Thyme

Insomnia
- Cedarwood
- Chamomile
- Clary Sage
- Lavender
- Marjoram
- Neroli
- Patchouli
- Sandalwood
- Valerian
- Ylang Ylang

Muscle Cramps
- Chamomile
- Eucalyptus
- Geranium
- Lavender
- Lemon
- Lime
- Marjoram
- Oregano
- Peppermint

Nausea
- Basil
- Coriander
- Cinnamon
- Dill
- Eucalyptus
- Fennel
- Frankincense
- Ginger
- Grapefruit
- Lavender
- Marjoram
- Myrrh
- Orange
- Peppermint
- Rosemary

- Thyme

Shock
- Clary sage
- Lavender
- Mandarin
- Neroli
- Peppermint
- Rose
- Ylang Ylang

Sore throat
- Cinnamon
- Cypress
- Eucalyptus
- Frankincense
- Geranium
- Lavender
- Lemon
- Marjoram
- Myrrh
- Oregano
- Peppermint
- Sandalwood
- Tea Tree
- Thyme

Respiratory Problems

- Basil
- Bergamot
- Chamomile
- Clary Sage
- Lemon
- Rosemary

Toothache

- Birch
- Cinnamon
- Clove
- Eucalyptus
- Frankincense
- Lavender
- Lemon
- Peppermint
- Rosemary
- Tea Tree

Conclusion

Thank you again for purchasing this book!

I hope it was able to provide you with all the information you need to help you to introduce Essential Oils into your life.

The next step is to purchase a few oils and start practicing using them on mild health problems to help you to gain confidence in your use of oils.

Below are 7 of the most commonly used oils to get you started:

- Eucalyptus

- Frankincense

- Lavender

- Lemon

- Peppermint

- Tea Tree

- Ylang Ylang

Once you have got used to using the oils, why not attempt some of the recipes in the book and make yourself a few healthy treats for your skin.

Finally, if you enjoyed this book, then I'd like to ask you for a favor, would you be kind enough to leave a review for this book on Amazon? It'd be greatly appreciated!

Thank you and good luck!

www.ingramcontent.com/pod-product-compliance
Lightning Source LLC
Chambersburg PA
CBHW050810290526
45792CB00001B/56